Janderson Castro dos Santos

Evidence-Based Implant Dentistry

Janderson Castro dos Santos

# Evidence-Based Implant Dentistry

Implant geometry, selection of grafting materials
and prevention of operative complications

ScienciaScripts

**Imprint**

Any brand names and product names mentioned in this book are subject to trademark, brand or patent protection and are trademarks or registered trademarks of their respective holders. The use of brand names, product names, common names, trade names, product descriptions etc. even without a particular marking in this work is in no way to be construed to mean that such names may be regarded as unrestricted in respect of trademark and brand protection legislation and could thus be used by anyone.

Cover image: www.ingimage.com

This book is a translation from the original published under ISBN 978-3-330-75676-2.

Publisher:
Sciencia Scripts
is a trademark of
Dodo Books Indian Ocean Ltd. and OmniScriptum S.R.L publishing group

120 High Road, East Finchley, London, N2 9ED, United Kingdom
Str. Armeneasca 28/1, office 1, Chisinau MD-2012, Republic of Moldova, Europe
Printed at: see last page
**ISBN: 978-620-8-28095-6**

# SUMMARY

# CHAPTER I. BIOMECHANICAL AND GEOMETRIC ASPECTS THAT CAN INFLUENCE THE SUCCESS OF SHORT DENTAL IMPLANTS

Janderson Castro dos Santos1 Ubiratan Santos Carvalho2 Heberte Cavalcante Abreu3

1- Graduated in Dentistry ITPAC Araguaína-TO, Master in Dentistry São Leopoldo Mandic Campinas-SP, Specialist in Implant Dentistry FACIT, Araguaína-TO. 2- Graduated in Dentistry ITPAC Araguaína-TO, Specialist in Implant Dentistry FACIT Araguaína-TO 3- Master's degree in Dentistry - concentration area in Oral and Maxillofacial Surgery UNIMAR, Marilia SP, PhD student in Implant Dentistry at the Dental Research Center - São Leopoldo Mandic Campinas SP, Coordinator of the Specialization Course in Oral and Maxillofacial Surgery and Traumatology and Professor of the Specialization Course in Implant Dentistry FACIT, Araguaína-TO.

## Summary

This is a non-systematic literature review designed to gather current technical scientific data to help make decisions when recommending short implants. Using the keyword 'short implants' on the Google Scholar search engine, a total of 18 free-circulation articles published between 2000 and 2016 were selected, including systematic or non-systematic literature reviews and clinical trials that address the success rate of short implants. Data regarding biomechanical aspects, micro and macro geometry that may influence current success rates were also reviewed. The average success rate found in this review was 94.30%, with the lowest being 85.65% and the highest 100%. As for the aspects that can negatively influence the success rate, the inadequate implant/crown ratio and the low bone quality of the implant site were the aspects that were most warned against, while positive influences were attributed to surface treatment as it contributes to stability along with large diameter implants, conical geometry and cervical micro-spirals were advocated as they minimize the risk of peri-implant bone loss.

**Key words:** Short implants, implant geometry, implant-crown ratio.

## 1- Introduction

The use of osseointegrated implants has become more popular over the years and every day more people are seeking out this specialty to solve functional and aesthetic problems related to tooth loss. The success rate of osseointegrated implants is well known and currently shows results of over 80% in oral rehabilitations with conventional implants or implants longer than 10 mm (Silva et al.[1] 2015).

The appropriate indication of osseointegrated implants depends on factors related to the quantity and quality of bone that the region to receive the implant must have, so that at the time of installation primary stability is achieved by locking the implant in close contact with the surgical bed and consequently the phenomenon of bone integration is achieved in accordance with the period necessary for complete healing (Camargo et al.[2] 2015).

In the daily routine of implant dentists, the majority of patients who seek rehabilitative care with implants have suffered tooth loss for more than 5 years and as a result are often in an advanced state of physiological resorption of the alveolar bone, implying a reduction in the height and thickness of the bone needed to install implants.

The maxillary bone is extremely porous and tooth loss in the posterior region causes resorption of the alveolar bone both vertically and horizontally. Due to the pressure differences caused by breathing in the maxillary sinus, pneumatization of the maxillary sinus can also occur along with the bone remodeling process, making it impossible to indicate conventional length implants. In cases where there is a great deal of bone loss in the vertical direction in the posterior region of the maxilla, surgery to elevate the floor of the maxillary sinus is generally indicated. The addition of grafting procedures to implant treatment, although proven to be effective, has the disadvantage of generating greater patient fear, adding to financial costs and increasing the time needed to recover and complete the treatment (Buringo, Martins[3] 2015).

When missing teeth occur in the lower arch, the delay in seeking rehabilitative treatment with implants also causes certain limitations due to the continuity of the alveolar bone resorption process that began after the extraction, causing the inferior alveolar nerve to be closer to the crestal surface, limiting bone height and thickness for the installation of conventional length implants without prior bone grafting procedures (Oliveira et al.[4] 2015).

In order to install implants in the posterior mandibular region with large vertical bone loss, the first option usually offered to patients is grafting and/or surgery to lateralize the inferior alveolar nerve. Although this procedure is effective, it is often limited by its high financial cost and the need for more time to recover and complete the treatment, causing greater anxiety and fear for patients who wish to go ahead with the treatment.

Short implants were developed with the aim of providing an alternative form of dental rehabilitation for patients with reduced bone height and making it possible to rehabilitate patients with atrophic jaws without the need for bone grafting procedures. Standard 7mm implants appeared in 1979, to be used alone or in conjunction with conventional-sized implants. However, the fact that they did not have characteristics different from long implants that compensated for their reduced size meant that high failure rates were reported in studies published in the 1980s and 1990s, which argued against their use (Romero et al.[5] 2006).

Advances in contemporary studies in the field of bioengineering have contributed to improving the success rate and safety in the indication of short implants. Changes in the morphology of current implants, as well as the discovery of the importance of secondary stability, new surface treatment techniques, the emergence of implants with different thread patterns, different geometries and increased diameters, are characteristics that have been linked to an increase of up to 300% in bone-implant contact, making it increasingly possible to achieve success when indicating rehabilitations with short implants. (Chag et al.[6] 2012, Borges et al.[7] 2013).

The aim of this non-systematic review of the literature is to collect current scientific technical data that will contribute to decision-making when indicating short implants as a viable, more accessible and less invasive alternative for the rehabilitation of missing dental elements.

## 2-Review of the Literature

Santiago et al.[8] (2010), with the aim of discussing the characteristics and indications of short implants considering biomechanical aspects, carried out a literature review in which they analyzed 69 articles published between 1990 and 2009, including clinical, laboratory and review studies that emphasized the length of osseointegrated implants. The studies were classified into levels of evidence and the searches were filtered, resulting in only 26 articles which were taken into account when drawing up the results. The results of the evaluation of the studies showed that short implants are a predictable treatment option in order to avoid invasive procedures such as bone grafts or lateralization of the inferior alveolar nerve. Most of the studies evaluated mentioned that implant geometry such as diameter, shape, thread pattern and surface treatment are compensatory factors for the short implant length. The bone quality of the surgical site is a factor that should be well assessed in surgical planning, and single implants should be avoided, opting for splinting between the implants in order to better dissipate masticatory forces along the long axis of the implant.

Sànchez-Garcés et al.[9] (2010), in a descriptive study, evaluated the performance of 273 short implants, measuring between 5 and 10 mm, installed in regions with severe alveolar resorption. The follow-up period ranged from 18 months to 12 years (mean 81 months). In this study, the type of surface, location and length of the implant were evaluated. The overall survival rate was 92.67%. When 10 mm implants were compared with smaller implants, survival rates were 92.82% and 92.5%, respectively. The highest number of failures was observed in relation to the surface of the implants: machined implants had a lower survival rate (5.9%) than surface-treated implants (8.9%). The posterior region of the maxilla also had a higher failure rate than the posterior mandible, with anterior regions showing no significant differences.

Galvâo el al.[10] (2011) carried out a non-systematic literature review in order to address biomechanical aspects, success rates, longevity and surgical and prosthetic planning of dental implants with a length of less than 10 mm. For this study, journal articles on short implants published between 2000 and 2009 were analyzed. Analysis of the studies reviewed shows that the success rate of short implants is between 79.3% and 92%, resulting in an average rate of 85.65%. The highest success rates were achieved when surface-treated implants were installed in type II bone regions, showing that surface treatment depends on bone quality to achieve greater success. When evaluating biomechanical aspects, they concluded that the diameter of the implants has a greater influence than the length on the dissipation of forces and tensions caused by chewing, as the region that receives the most tension is located closest to the bone crest. The splinting of crowns in the planning of prosthetic crowns with a proportion compatible with the length of the implant, the adoption of a reduced occlusal table, the non-use of cantilevers favor biomechanics and increase the predictability of treatment.

Chang et al.[6] (2011) carried out a study simulating the biomechanical behavior of short activated implants. They used finite element models constructed from computed tomography. The implants were 6 mm long and varied in diameter, being 6 mm, 7 mm or 8 mm. They were placed in bones of three qualities, from normal to osteoporotic. No statistically significant results were obtained for vertical loads, i.e. the reduced length did not result in greater or lesser bone pressure capable of compromising the peri-implant tissues. Under lateral loads, the force increased by 58.58% in implants placed in poor bone (6 mm in diameter). In larger diameter implants (7 mm or 8 mm) the strength increased by around 52%. Therefore, in a case that develops in this way, the ideal way to minimize possible losses is to use the largest diameter implants possible.

The geometric shape of implants in general has changed over the years and the most commonly used implant-crown connection was the external hexagon, which has gradually been replaced by the Morse Cone connection. Cone Morse implants have shown greater advantages when compared to other types of crown/implant connection. Among these, the possibility of the crown/implant junction being located intrasulcularly and far from the bone crest reduces the rate of peri-implant bone loss through biological isolation, provides better distribution of masticatory stresses, gives greater resistance to eccentric stresses and bending, resulting in greater prosthetic stability (Pellizzer & Carvalho[11] 2011).

Menchero-Catalejo et al.[12] (2011) monitored 2087 implants with a length of 10 mm or less, used in oral rehabilitation with limited bone availability. After ten years of clinical and radiographic follow-up, the results were similar between long implants with a success rate of 92.5% and short implants with a treated surface with a success rate of 98.42%. According to the authors, the surface treatment of the implants was undoubtedly one of the factors that proved the successes found in rehabilitations involving short implants.

Annibali et al[13] . (2012) conducted a study to evaluate the success rate of short implants in atrophic mandibles. Biological (individual health) and biomechanical (prosthesis function) complications were taken into account, along with marginal (peri-implant) bone loss. Two controlled studies and 14 observational studies were selected for data collection, totaling 6193 short implants inserted in 3848 patients. The results of the analysis indicated a biological success rate of 98.8% and a biomechanical success rate of 99.4%. Taking into account the average observation time of two years, the success rate of short implants was 99.1%.

Urdaneta et al.[14] (2012) Conducted a retrospective study with approximately two years of follow-up. For this study, 410 short (8 mm) and ultra-short (6 mm and 5 mm) implants (Bicon®) were installed to monitor survival rates. Of the total sample, 322 were restored with single crowns and 163 implants were installed in the posterior mandibular region. During follow-up, nine implants were lost, four 8 mm and five 6 mm, no 5 mm implants were lost, there were no statistically significant differences between short and ultra-short implants and the success rate was 99.55%. Of the failures that occurred, seven were reported before prosthetic loading, and two were splinted prostheses. It was concluded that the predictability of ultra-short implants is similar to that of short implants.

The study by Lops et al.[15] (2012) followed 121 patients from the Dental Department of the University of Milan (Italy) for 20 years, in which 257 implants were installed, 108 of which were 8 mm long and 149 of which were 10 mm long. The survival rate was 92.3% for 8 mm implants and 95.9% for 10 mm implants, giving a total of 94.1%. The authors confirmed the high success rate of short implants in prosthetic rehabilitation, and the prognosis shown in the posterior region was 95%, similar to that found in the anterior region, with a value of 96.4%.

Pellizzer et al.[16] (2013) based on the pre-supposition established in the literature where many authors mention that the main disadvantage of short implants is the possibility of vertical cantilever formation generated by the disproportion in the implant crown ratio, a test was carried out to evaluate the distribution of stresses in the peri-implant bone tissue in short 8.5 mm implants, with a diameter of 4.0 mm and a cone-Morse prosthetic connection, with crown heights of 10.0 mm and 15.00 mm, under axial and oblique loads. The evaluation was carried out 'ex vivo' in which two models were made using the programs Invesalius 3.0,

Rhinoceros 4.0 and Solidworks 2010. These models consisted of a bone block with a short (3.75 x 8.5 mm) Morse cone implant inserted. The height of the crown (cemented) was set at 10.00 mm and 15.00 mm. The models were processed using the Femap 10 and NeiNastran 10.0 programs and then 200N (vertical) and 100N (oblique) forces were applied in different directions. The results showed that the length of crowns retained on short implants is detrimental to the peri-implant tissue, thus representing an important step in the proper planning of implant-supported prostheses The distal and mesial regions showed the highest concentration of stresses under oblique loading. Oblique loading was the most damaging when compared to axial loading, and was statistically significant.

Borges et al.[7] (2013) in a literature review analyzed articles published between 200 and 2012 that referred to the success rate of short implants and observed that the success rate found in this period was between 88% and 100%. Among the studies analyzed, the one with the lowest success rate (88%) was published in 2000 and evaluated 68 implants measuring 7.0 and 8.0 mm in length installed in the mandibular bone and followed up over a period of 8 years, while the study with the highest cumulative success rate (100%) was published in 2004. The sample included 168 implants measuring 6.0 and 8.0 mm in length, of which 128 were rehabilitated with single crowns and 40 with fixed prostheses, both installed in the maxilla and mandible and followed up for 6.5 years. As for the main aspects highlighted for influencing the success rate, they reported that surface treatment with acid etching and sandblasting was superior to implants with surfaces treated by titanium plasma spray. Poor bone quality, occlusal overload and infections were the main factors related to failure.

Manfro et al.[17] (2013) carried out a case-control study in which they followed up four consecutive cases of severely resorbed mandibles for a period of 36 months and treated them with 7.5 to 10 mm long implants and protocol prostheses. The patients included in the study were females aged between 59 and 70 who underwent bone analysis using panoramic radiography and cone-beam computed tomography, resulting in an average alveolar ridge height of 7.0 mm. After installing the implants, the cases were re-evaluated at 7, 15, 30, 60, 90 and 180 days, where they were observed for the clinical and radiographic peri-implant situation and the stability of the prostheses was checked. Based on the items evaluated, the success rate obtained at the end of the evaluation period was 94.12%. The average peri-implant bone loss was 0.71mm, considered within the normal range for external hexagon implants with conventional platforms.

Queiroz et al[18] (2014) carried out a clinical study to compare the survival rate between short implants and implants with a length of 10 mm or more. For this analysis, 48 short implants

(5.5 mm x 5 mm / 7 mm x 5 mm) were compared to 42 long implants (10 mm x 4 mm / 11.5 mm x 4 mm) using the resonance frequency analysis method to quantify the osseointegration values. Of the implants in the sample, six short implants were lost, resulting in an 87.5% survival rate, while the long implants had a 100% survival rate. Despite this result, the author considers the use of short implants in atrophic posterior mandibles to be an applicable alternative.

Rossi et al.[19] (2015), in order to verify the success rate of short implants, installed 40 SLActive® implants (Straumann) 6 mm high in posterior regions, and after six weeks, single porcelain crowns were installed. The authors evaluated an average marginal bone loss rate of 0.7 ± 0.6 mm and 100% implant survival after prosthetic loading. It was concluded that short implants with a moderately rough surface in posterior regions showed a highly favorable behavior, with no loss in up to five years of follow-up.

Michel et al.[20] (2015) analyzed relevant studies published between 2004 and 2015 and found that the survival rate of short implants ranged from 89.3% to 100%, resulting in a mean value of 94.65%. It is important to note that the lowest success rates reported were in studies published in 1990, where there was no concern about implant surface treatment and the implants used had a reduced diameter of 3.5 mm. Even with limitations relating to the geometry of some implants in the sample, the authors considered the use of short implants to be feasible. The studies that achieved the highest success rates were those published recently (2015) where the implants submitted for evaluation had different morphologies with a length of 6.0 mm but a diameter of more than 3.5 mm, as well as treated surfaces. As for the biomechanical aspects that interfere with success rates, discussions have been raised about the implant crown relationship, implant site bone density, correct occlusal adjustment for the distribution of masticatory loads, implant diameter. Concerns about the implant crown ratio have been reduced with the emergence of claims that the implant crown ratio does not resemble the root crown ratio and that the success of short implants depends more on the correct occlusal fit than on the implant crown ratio.

Gonçalves et al.[21] (2015) found divergences in the criteria used to evaluate the results provided by articles on the clinical performance of short implants and carried out a systematic review in order to emphasize the essential parameters needed to characterize the long-term clinical success of short and extra-short implants. For this systematic review, articles published between March 2000 and February 2014 were analyzed by two reviewers based on standardized inclusion criteria. Only articles with a clear objective of investigating the long-term performance of implants with a length of less than 10 mm installed in humans, studies that clearly described the criteria for characterizing failures, with a minimum sample of 10 implants followed up for a minimum period of one year after the application of occlusal loads were included. A total of 1174 studies were evaluated, of which only 13 provided information on the 24 pre-established parameters. The most frequently evaluated parameters among the total number of studies evaluated were marginal bone loss, cumulative implant survival rate, followed by implant failure rate and biological complications such as bleeding on probing and probing depth. The results of the analysis of the eligible studies showed that short implants are a successful treatment option with cumulative success rates of between 84% and 100% in studies with a follow-up of between 5 and 10 years, resulting in an average of 92%.

Pereira et al.[22] (2015) conducted a study to compare the behavior of four types of implants (Implacil De Bortoli, São Paulo/SP, Brazil) with different geometries:

• Cylindrical implant with external hexagonal connection (CIL HE): made up of a cylindrical body, self-tapping conical apex, external hexagonal connection and smooth 1.8mm cervical collar in a slightly divergent (conical) shape;

• Cylindrical implant with internal hexagonal connection (CIL HI): made up of a cylindrical body, self-tapping conical apex, internal hexagonal connection and smooth 1.8mm cervical collar in a slightly divergent (conical) shape;

• Conical implant with internal hexagonal connection (CON HI): made up of a conical-shaped body, internal hexagonal connection, micro-threads in the cervical region and a smooth 1 mm collar;

• Conical implant with external hexagonal connection (CON HE): made up of a conical-shaped body, external hexagonal connection, micro-threads in the cervical region and a 1 mm flat collar.

The study included patients rehabilitated with implant-supported fixed prostheses in function for at least 1 year at the Dentistry Center of the University of São Paulo (USP) between 1998 and 2012.

resulting in a total of 183 patients (69 men and 114 women), rehabilitated with 938 implants. The results showed a mean marginal bone loss of cylindrical implants of (2.29 ± 1.16 mm), which was higher than that of conical implants (1.91 ± 1.22 mm), resulting in statistically significant differences (P<0.001). Implant geometry and smooth collar length have a significant influence on peri-implant bone loss. Tapered implants, with cervical micro-spirals and shorter smooth collar length, showed less marginal bone loss.

## 2.1 Correlation of pre-existing results in the reviewed literature.

Based on the principle that the approach to decision-making in the health area should use the best available evidence, in line with the patient's wishes, we carried out a comparative analysis of success rates and qualitative data relating to short implants in order to raise hypotheses to guide the best clinical decision (Faber[23] 2008).

### 2.1.1 Nomeclaturas

With regard to nomenclature, there was broad agreement among the authors reviewed that implants with a length of less than 10 mm are considered short. However, Michel et al.[20] (2015), Undaneta et al.[14] (2012) have mentioned that there is a category of even smaller implants called extra short or ultra short implants with a length varying between 6.0 and 4.0 mm. The 4.0 mm implant is the smallest dental implant currently available on the market and is manufactured by the Swiss company Straumann.

According to the consensus on implant success, survival and failure, the success rate, as an ideal result, was evaluated by the absence of mobility, bone loss of less than 2 mm, with reference to the initial radiograph after surgery, absence of previous exudate and pain. Some authors have presented a success rate based on the survival rate of implants, for which the evaluation criteria are less rigorous, where radiographic bone loss can reach up to 4 mm, according to the initial radiograph. However, this bone loss acts differently in a short implant, as 4 mm can characterize its failure rate in implants smaller than 8.0 mm. Manfro et al.[17] (2013), Rossi et al.[19] (2015) attributed success to implants with a length of less than 8.0 mm where marginal bone loss was between 0.71 mm and approximately 0.6 mm respectively.

### 2.1.2 An opinion on the indication of short implants based on literature review studies.

Different types of studies have been reviewed in this writing, including non-systematic literature reviews in order to gather data on the success rates of short implants, Galvâo et al.[10] (2011), Borges et al.[7] (2013) reviewed articles published between 2000 and 2009, and 2000 and 20012 respectively, the success rate found in the review by Borges et al.[7] (2013) was between 88% and 100%, the lowest rate in the range is higher than the lowest rate in the range found in the study by Galvao et al.[10] (2011), which found rates between 79.3% and 92%.

Although the methodology used to evaluate the studies is not exactly the same to allow fair comparisons, the increase in the success rate of short implants has been remarkable and leads us to conclude that professional technical mastery has been improved. The combination of technical mastery and the technology applied to current implants has contributed positively to the longevity of short implants, allowing for safer indications based on up-to-date scientific evidence.

### 2.1.3 Results of clinical studies on the longevity of short implants.

Osseointegration is a phenomenon that undoubtedly occurs when nickel titanium implants are installed, regardless of their length or diameter, provided that primary instability has been achieved during the surgical stage. The notification of an intimate contact relationship between the implant surface and the bone tissue is one of the primary criteria indicative of success in implant dentistry. However, the greatest concern regarding short implants is based on the assumption that the smaller the implant, the less its capacity to resist masticatory forces over a long period of time, compromising the longevity of success when short implants are indicated.

In order to find out more about the longevity of success of short implants, retrospective studies were consulted for this article. Menchero-Catalejo et al.[12] (2011) followed up patients for a period of 10 years with implants starting at 10 mm in length and with treated surfaces, and obtained a success rate of 98.42%; lops et al.[15] (2012) demonstrated a longer follow-up period (20 years) in their study where the length of the implants analyzed was specified at 8 and 10 mm, achieving a success rate of 95.9%; Undaneta et al.[14] (2012), specified the length of the implants at 5, 6 and 8 mm, followed up for a period of 2 years and obtained a success rate of 99.55%. The comparative analysis of these studies allows us to understand that short implants have been shown to last in acceptable clinical conditions for long periods of time, with little reduction in the success rate over the years, especially when the implants have been professionally monitored.

The degree of relevance of the success rates is directly related to the number of implants, length and follow-up time. Figure 1 was drawn up in order to make a comparative analysis between the studies based on these criteria.

| Clinical studies | (N) Quantity Implants | Implant length in mm | Time of Follow-up | success rate |
|---|---|---|---|---|
| **Sanchez-Garcés et al. (2010)** | 273 | Between 5.0 and 10 | 18 months to 12 years | 92,67% |
| **Menchero-Catalejo et al. (2011)** | 2087 | ≤10 | 10 years | 98,4% |
| **Undaneta et al. (2012)** | 410 | 8,0 - 6,0 - 5,0 | 2 years | 99,55% |

| Lops et al. (2012) | 257 | 8,0 e 10 | 20 years | 94,1% |
| *Queiroz et al. (2014) | 48 | 5,5 -7,0 | | 87,5% |
| Rossi et al. (2015) | 40 | 6,0 | 5 years | 100% |

Figure 1   - Ratio of success rate, sample, length and radiographic clinical follow-up time.

The study by Menchero-Catalejo et al.[12] (2011) presented the largest sample of implants evaluated (2087), which consisted of implants with a length of 10 mm or less, followed up for a period of 10 years, resulting in a success rate of 98.4%, Sanchez-Garcés et al.[9] (2010) evaluated a smaller number of implants (273) with the same lengths, but followed them up for a longer period of time (12 years), resulting in a slightly lower success rate of 92.67% (see figure 1). When we look at the follow-up time, we see that the longer period had a slightly lower success rate; however, this reduction does not compromise the effectiveness of short implants, allowing us to consider them a viable treatment alternative.

In the most recent studies, Undaneta et al.[14] (2012) and Rossi et al.[19] (2015) only included implants shorter than 10 mm in their sample, which were followed up for a period of 2 and 5 years and achieved success rates of 99.55% and 100% respectively, when compared to the study by lops et al.[15] (2012), who followed up for 20 years (94.1%), we are led to assume that the length of time that short implants have been in service reduces the success rate a little, showing that short implants demonstrate longevity, making their indication safe when submitted to adequate clinical and radiographic follow-up (see figure 1).

When we compare the results of the clinical studies shown in figure 1, we note that *Queiroz et al.[18] (2014) had a lower success rate and no follow-up time for the cases evaluated. The omission of the follow-up time and the low success rate of *Queiroz et al.[18] (2014) (87.5%) is related to the different methodological resource, which was based on resonance frequency to quantify the osseointegration values, which nevertheless does not invalidate its clinical indication.

### 2.1.4 Different aspects that influence clinical success when using short implants.

Although Santiago et al.[8] (2010) did not focus their review on providing quantitative data on the success rate of implants, they have provided qualitative data by pointing out that the macro and micro geometry of short implants was already a subject of discussion in the period between 1990 and 2000, where they reported that the geometry and thread pattern had a significant influence on clinical success in order to compensate for the reduced length of the implant. Pereira et al.[22] (2015) evaluated long and short implants and found that tapered implants with cervical micro-spirals and shorter smooth collar lengths showed less marginal bone loss.

There is agreement between Santiago et al.[8] (2010), Galvao et al.[10] (2011) and Borges et al.[7] (2013) regarding the indication of crown splinting in order to avoid axial overloads, which is one of the main factors compromising the longevity of short implants.

Biomechanical aspects are extremely important factors in maintaining the stability of short implants Chang et al.[6] (2011) and Pellizer et al.[16](2013) carried out laboratory tests simulating the masticatory forces applied to the implants to assess the possible damage they could cause to the peri-implant tissues. Both authors, although using different methodologies, revealed that axial loads are less damaging than oblique loads, and also reported that the use of implants with a wider diameter is indicated to minimize peri-implant bone loss. The disproportionate crown-to-implant relationship was a factor emphasized by the authors in order to avoid the formation of vertical cantilevers which induce bone resorption, especially in the mesial and distal areas of the implants, putting longevity at risk.

Pellizzer, Carvalho[11] (2011) mention that implants with an internal Morse Cone connection minimize marginal bone loss and promote better propagation of masticatory forces along the long axis of the implants. However, the indication of these implants requires infraosseous installation, a fact that sometimes limits their indication in bone beds that are limited in the vertical direction.

Surface treatment has been mentioned positively as it contributes to better success rates, but it must be combined with adequate bone quality (type II density) in order to achieve greater success (Galvâo et al.[10] .2011), Menchero Catalejo et al.[12] (2011) reported that short implants with treated surfaces (98.42%) had higher success rates than implants of conventional length (92.5%).

Borges et al.[7] (2013) mentions that the type of surface treatment can influence the success rate, stating that acid etching and sandblasting is superior to the application of titanium plasma spray. The coarse-grained sandblasted and acid-etched SLA® (Sandblasted, Large-grit, Acid-etched) surface has become one of the best-documented roughened surfaces in implant dentistry and has demonstrated several advantages when compared to other surface treatments. The SLA® surface has proved successful on Straumann implants of different designs: narrow collar implants, wide collar implants, conical implants and short implants.

**2.1.5 Average success rate of short implants based on the articles reviewed.**

This review was made up of free-circulation articles published between 2010 and June 2016 found using the keyword 'short implants' in the Google Scholar search. A total of 18 articles made up this non-systematic review, of which 12 presented quantitative data on the success rate of short implants and 6 provided only qualitative data on the aspects that can influence the success rate. Among the articles reviewed, the systematic review by Galvâo et al.[10] (2015) mentioned that the success rate of short implants is around 92%. Considering this data together with the other articles reviewed, the present study found an overall average of 94.30%, a higher rate than that of Galvâo et al.[10] (2015). This superiority may be related to the inclusion of recent articles in this review, as well as the inclusion criteria of articles based on less systematic criteria (see Figure 2).

| Author and year of publication | index of Success % |
|---|---|
| Sanchez-Garcés et al. (2010) | 92,67 |
| Menchero-Catalejo et al. (2011 ) | 98,42 |
| Galvâo el al. (2011) | 85,65 |
| Undaneta et al. (2012) | 99,5 |
| Lops et al (2012) | 94,1 |
| Annibali et al (2012) | 99,1 |
| Manfro et al. (2013) | 94,12 |
| Borges et al. 2013 | 94,0 |
| Queiroz et al (2014) | 87,5 |
| Rossi et al (2015) | 100 |
| Michel et al (2015) | 94,65 |
| Gonçalves et al, (2015) | 92,0 |
| Total | **94,30%** |

**Figure 2- Overall average success rate found in this literature review**

**3-Conclusion**

•	The average success rate for short implants found in this study was 94.30%, showing that short implants are viable alternatives for rehabilitation in areas of severe bone resorption;

• The implant-to-bone ratio was a much-discussed aspect among the authors, proving to be the major villain, along with the bone quality of the implant site, which should be well assessed when planning using short implants;

• Occlusal adjustment must be carried out thoroughly in order to avoid excessive overloads that could compromise implant stability during masticatory function;

• Crown splinting is recommended to provide greater resistance to masticatory forces and consequently promotes a reduction in peri-implant bone loss.

• In terms of geometry, larger diameter implants provide greater stability for prostheses with increased implant-bone contact; conical shaped implants with cervical micro-spirals and a narrow metal collar minimize marginal bone loss,

• The different surface treatment techniques have had a positive influence on the current success rates of short implants, providing greater predictability.

**4-References·**

1.    Silva BCR, Carvalho PSP, Vedovato O, Bassi APS, Conforte JJ, Ponzoni D. Retrospective study of the survival rate of implants installed by professionals with different degrees of experience in implant dentistry. RFO, Passo Fundo. 2015: 20(3): 295-301.

2.    Camargo BA, Tres M, Spazzi AO, Magagnin C, Schuh C. Influence of milling techniques on the primary stability of osseointegrated implants - an in vitro study. Full Dent. Sci. 2015; 6(22):160-l64.

3.    Buringo JB, Martins FR. Maxillary sinus lift with biomaterial as late implant preparation. Revista UNIPLAC. 2015; 3(1) 22-27.

4.    Oliveira MM, Terra GAP, Coêlho TMK, Masocatto DC, Gaetti-Jardim EC, Destefani MS, Hassumi JS. Rehabilitation of atrophic posterior mandible using the inferior alveolar nerve transposition technique associated with implant installation. Arch Health Invest. 2015; 4(4): 1-6.

5.    Romeo E, MD, Ghisolfi M, Rozza R, Chiapasco M, Lops D. Short (8-mm) Dental Implants in the Rehabilitation of Partial and Complete Edentulism: A 3- to 14-Year Longitudinal Study Int J Prosthodont 2006; 19(5):586-592.

6.    Chang, SH, Lin CL, Hsue SS, Lin YS, et al. Biomechanical analysis of the effects of implant diameter and bone quality in short implants placed in the atrophic posterior maxilla.

---

J. Med Eng Phys. 2012; 34(2):153-6o.

7.    Borges TF, Vaz RR, Barros VM, Rosa RM, Jùnior LMO. Clinical Performance Using Short Implants: Literature Review. UNOPAR Cient Ciênc Biol Saùde 2013; 5(4):311 -7.

8.    Santiago Jûnior JF, Verri, FR, Pellizzer EP, Moraes SLD, Carvalho BMC. Short dental implants: a conservative alternative for oral rehabilitation. Rev. Cir. Traumatol. Buco-Maxilo-fac. 2010; 10 (2): 67-76.

9.    Sànchez-Garcés M. A., Costa-Berenguer X., Gay-Escoda C. Short Implants: a descriptive study of 273 implants. Clin Implant Dent Relat Res, 2010 Oct 26: 1-9.

10.    Galvao FFSA, Almeida-Jûnior AA, Faria-Jûnior NB, Caldas SGFR, Reis JMSN, Margonar R. Predictability of short implants: literature review. RSBO. 2011 Jan-Mar;8(1):81-8.

11.    Pellizzer EP ,Carvalho PSP. Fundamentals of implant dentistry: a contemporary view. Sao Paulo: Quintessence, 2011.

12.    Menchero-Cantalejo E, Barona-Dorado C, Cantero-Alvarez, M, Fernândez-Câliz F, Martinez-Gonzâlez JM. Meta-analysis on the survival of short implants. Med Oral Pathol Oral Cir Bucal 2011;16(4):546-51.

13.    Annibali, S. Short dental implants: a systematic review. J Dent Res, 2012: 91(1): 25-32.

14.    Urdaneta RA, Daher S, Leary J, Emanuel KM, Chuang SK. The survival of ultrashort locking-taper implants. Int J Oral Maxillofac Implants 2012; 27(3):644-54

15.    Lops D, Bressan E, Pisoni G, Cea N, Corazza B, Romeo E. Short implants in partially edentuolous maxillae and mandibles: a 10 to 20 years retrospective evaluation. International J Dent. 2012; Article ID 351793, doi:10.1155/2012/351793.1-8.

16.    Pellizzer EP, Moraes SLD, Santiago Junior JF, Almeida DAF, Honório HM, Ramos Verri FR. Short Morse cone implants: crown-to-implant ratio. Rev. Cir. Traumatol. Buco-Maxilo-Fac. 2013; 13 (3): 79-86

17.    Manfro R, Bortoluzzi MC, Pratto LM, Fabris V, Cecconello R, Bitencourt AZ. Severely Resorbed Edentulous Mandibles Treated with Short Implants Presentation of 4 Clinical Cases and 30 to 36 Month Control J Oral Invest. 2013: 2(1): 10-16.

18.    Queiroz TP, Aguiar SC, Margonar R, Souza Faloni AP, Gruber R, Luvizuto ER. Clinical study on survival rate of short implants placed in the posterior mandibular region: resonance frequency analysis. Clin Oral Implants Res 2014; 12(9):1-7.

19.   Rossi F, Lang NP, Ricci E, Ferraioli L, Marchetti C, Botticelli D. Early loading of 6-mm-short implants with a moderately rough surface supporting single crowns - a prospective 5-year cohort study. Clin Oral Implants Res 2015; 26(4):471-7.

20.   Michel RC, Damante CA, Rezende MLR, Sant'ana ACPS, Greghi SLA, Zangrando MSR. Predictability of single-unit short and extra-short implants in an atrophic posterior mandible. RFO, Passo Fundo 2015; 20 (2): 258-263.

21.   Gonçalves TMSV, Bortolini S, Martinolli M, Alfenas BFM, Peruzzo DC, Natali A, Berzaghi A, Cunha R, Garcia MR. Long-term Short Implants Performance: Systematic Review and Meta-Analysis of the Essential Assessment Parameters. Brazilian Dental Journal (2015) 26(4): 325-336.

22.   Pereira MA. The influence of implant geometry on peri-implant bone loss: a cross-sectional study in humans. [Master's dissertation]. Florianópolis: Federal University of Santa Catarina Health Sciences Center;2015.

23.   Faber J. Evidence-based dentistry: the foundation of clinical decision-making. R Dentai Press Ortodon Ortop Facial (2008) 13 (01): 5.

# CHAPTER II. MAXILLARY SINUS LIFT: BIOMATERIAL SELECTION CRITERIA

Janderson Castro dos Santos1 Cristiano Prado Coelho2

1- Graduated in Dentistry ITPAC Araguaína-TO, Specialist in Implant Dentistry FACIT Araguaína-TO, Master in Dentistry São Leopoldo Mandic Campinas-SP. 2- Graduated in Dentistry, Specialist in Implant Dentistry FACIT Araguaína-TO

## Summary

The loss of teeth in the posterior region of the maxilla and the patient's advancing age result in resorption of the alveolar bone and subsequent pneumatization of the maxillary sinuses, which often makes it impossible to install implants without involving a grafting procedure. The surgical procedure of elevating the floor of the maxillary sinus is the treatment option available to enable rehabilitation with implants in these situations. Different grafting materials have been mentioned in the literature as viable options for carrying out this procedure, offering professionals a wide choice of materials that can be used. The aim of this literature review study is to highlight the main advantages and disadvantages of the main grafting materials mentioned in the literature in order to gather scientific technical data to help professionals choose the most suitable grafting material for this procedure. Articles on the subject were consulted and classified according to their origin: autogenous, homogenous, xenogenous and alloplastic for later comparison. In most of the articles reviewed, it can be concluded that autogenous grafts are still considered the gold standard. However, the characteristics of bovine xenografts (*Bio-Oss®* (Geistlich Biomaterials, Wolhusen, CH Switzerland), even though they do not have osteogenic capacity, have shown satisfactory results, as well as a higher rate of maintenance of the grafted volume when compared to other materials. The properties of *Bio-Oss®* have made this material attractive, making it the material of choice among professionals when performing sinus lift surgery.

**Key words:** bone graft; maxillary sinus; biomaterials.

## 1    Introduction

The rate of tooth loss in the young adult population is still considered high. A recent survey revealed that Brazilians aged between 35 and 44 have around 44.7% of their teeth compromised[1] . Among the population that most seeks dental clinics in search of rehabilitative treatment, the young adult population stands out, as they are in a better financial position and have the potential to pay for dental rehabilitation with implants, as this service is rarely offered in the public network.

High success rates have been related to dental implants from various points of view: from a biological point of view, the phenomenon of osseointegration stands out; from an aesthetic point of view, the possibility of rehabilitating with independent dental crowns with an appearance as close to natural as possible; from a biomechanical point of view, greater prosthetic stability and the ability to adequately withstand masticatory forces, providing greater safety, comfort and longevity for implants when compared to conventional fixed prostheses.[2]

In addition to alveolar bone resorption, the loss of teeth in the posterior region of the maxilla and the individual's advancing age result in pneumatization of the maxillary sinuses. Pneumatization consists of the process of bone remodelling of the maxillary sinus walls, resulting in the overextension of the Schneiderian membrane inside the maxillary bone, reducing bone volume, which often makes it impossible to install implants without involving a grafting procedure.[3]

To enable the installation of implants in the posterior region of the maxilla with extensive resorption, two techniques for lifting the floor of the maxillary sinus are generally the solutions most used by dental surgeons: the approach using a bone window in the lateral wall and the alveolar approach. The choice of technique to be used is based on the remaining residual bone structure and how much lifting of the floor will be required. After access with disruption of the inferior or anterolateral sinus wall, the Schneiderian membrane is detached and a space is created below between the membrane and the inferior wall, where it is grafted and/or implanted with bone from autogenous or allogenic sources, biomaterials or a combination of these materials.[2,4]

The literature describes that maxillary sinus lift procedures are required when the height of the residual bone below the sinus cavity is less than the ideal implant length required for prosthetic rehabilitation. Due to the limited bone volume of intraoral autogenous donor sites and the post-operative morbidity associated with autogenous grafts, alternative methods using synthetic bone, as well as fresh frozen allogeneic bone obtained from bone banks, represent an adequate, quick and less morbid supply for maxillo-mandibular reconstructions for implant rehabilitation.[5]

Among the various grafting materials, autogenous bone is recognized as the gold standard. Autogenous bone grafts originate from various donor areas and can be prepared in different ways for use in sinus lift surgery. They can be used as graft blocks or ground into granules to be used individually or in combination with bone substitutes.[6]

Histological studies have shown bone neoformation in maxillary sinuses grafted exclusively with biomaterials, suggesting that there is no considerable bone loss around these *Bio-Oss®*

biomaterials (Geistlich Biomaterials, wolhusen, CH Switzerland).[7] The use of bone substitutes as grafting material in maxillary sinus lifts has the great advantage of facilitating surgery and eliminating morbidity in the donor area. However, these bone substitutes are expensive and in situations where a large volume of graft is required, the combination of autogenous bone and biomaterials is necessary.[8]

Knowing that there are several biomaterials indicated for grafting in maxillary sinus lift surgery, this non-systematic literature review aims to emphasize the main advantages and disadvantages of the main grafting materials mentioned in current studies on this subject.

## 2    Literature review

### 2.1  Maxillary bone resorption process

The maintenance of the alveolar crest of the maxillary bone is conditioned by the existence of the dental element inside the alveolus, which together with the fibers of the periodontal ligament transfer masticatory forces to the supporting periodontium, stimulating the physiological process of remodeling and maintenance of the periodontal bone structure. However, as a result of tooth loss, periodontal ligament fibers are also lost and bone traction stimuli are interrupted, reducing bone apposition stimuli, making the process of bone resorption more significant than apposition.[9]

The maxillary bone is a highly porous bone in which part of its strength comes from the dental elements that fill the interior of the maxillary alveoli, representing real pillars of strength when you consider that its interior houses the maxillary sinus, a pneumatic structure that forms part of the respiratory system. The maxillary sinuses can vary in volume and shape and are generally asymmetrical. They are pyramidal cavities made up of the following walls:[10]

•    **Anterior or anterolateral wall**: this is a convex shape excavated by the canine fossa, its outer portion is thin and its uppermost portion contains the infraorbital foramen;

•    **Posterior Wall**: this is the structure referring to the inner portion of the maxillary tuberosity;

•    **Inferior wall:** in adults, this structure is located below the nasal floor and at its lowest point it divides the alveolar processes of the molars and pre-molars;

•    **Medial wall:** convex inside the maxillary sinus and quite thin, it contains the communication hole called the ostium, which varies in diameter between 3 and 6 mm.

The inside of the maxillary sinus is lined by the Schneiderian membrane, which is a thin layer of ciliated, cuboidal or columnar pseudo-stratified respiratory epithelium that is in close contact with the periosteum of the inner walls and has the function of secreting mucus to moisten and warm the inhaled air, as well as participating in the regulation of nasal pressure during barometric variations.[3]

In the event of tooth loss, changes in pressure inside the maxillary sinus caused by breathing begin to influence the bone remodeling process, inducing the invagination of the sinus floor towards the empty alveoli, which is known as the maxillary sinus pneumatization process, which makes dental rehabilitation in the posterior region of the maxilla more complex, requiring bone grafting procedures to enable the installation of osseointegrated implants.[5]

## 2.2 Main surgical methods for elevating the floor of the maxillary sinus.

To enable rehabilitation in the posterior maxillary region, two techniques for lifting the floor of the maxillary sinus are commonly used: the approach using a bone window in the lateral wall and the alveolar approach. The choice of technique to be used is based on the residual bone structure remaining and how much lifting of the floor will be required to install the implants .[3]

Maxillary sinus floor elevation surgery using the lateral window technique is indicated when a bone height gain of between 5 and 12 mm is required and the alveolar remnant is less than 5 mm in the sub-sinusal region, the conservative technique with intra-alveolar access requires a minimum alveolar bone remnant of 5 mm and is indicated for gains of a maximum of 5 mm in height. In this technique, the bone graft is placed by breaking through the floor of the maxillary sinus where the membrane is detached from the inferior wall, creating a space between the membrane and the floor where it is grafted and/or implanted using autogenous bone, allogeneic bone, biomaterials or a combination of these .[8]

## 2.3 Description and classification of the main grafting materials indicated for maxillary sinus elevation.

The biomaterials used in the different surgical techniques for elevating the floor of the maxillary sinus can be classified according to their origin :[7]

• **Autogenous:** these are grafts obtained from the patient himself from intra- or extra-oral regions;

• **Allograft or homogenous graft:** these are grafts from human bone banks which are subjected to a freezing and dehydration or freezing and dehydration demineralization process.

- **Xenografts or heterogeneous grafts:** these are grafts that undergo the same process as allografts, but come from a different species.

- **Alloplastics:** these are synthetic materials used for implantation in living tissue, such as bioceramic polymers/hydroxyapatite, tricalcium phosphate and bioactive glasses.

### 2.3.1 Autogenous grafts.

Autogenous bone grafts are usually chosen as the first choice, either because of their efficiency, biosafety or ease of procurement. They are made up of tissues from the individual themselves and are the only bone graft to provide immunocompatible live bone cells, essential for osteogenesis, which is responsible for the proliferation of bone cells, so the more living cells that are transplanted, the more bone tissue will be formed. There are, however, disadvantages and risks to its use, such as the insufficient amount of graft from the donor area and the consequent need for another surgical intervention site, which leads to greater morbidity, patient discomfort and prolonged recovery time .[11]

Autogenous bone grafts offer the best results for repairing lost bone tissue, as they provide the ideal characteristics, such as mechanical resistance, viable osteoblasts and greater efficiency. However, there are disadvantages and risks to their use, such as the creation of a second surgical site, such as in the iliac crest, which is associated with morbidity, as well as the progressive loss of volume due to the high degree of resorption .[12]

Extraoral alternatives include the skullcap, tibia and iliac crest, and intraoral alternatives include the maxillary tuber, which is the most suitable donor region for removing bone tissue to repair small and medium bone losses. The tuber is a medullary bone that is easier to access and recover, and can be removed bilaterally. It is the most commonly used for filling in particulate form in small fenestrations during preparation for implant placement, in the maxillary sinus cavity and dental alveolus with the installation of immediate implants. 3[1]

The maxillary tuberosity has a considerable amount of cancellous bone, where foci of red marrow can be seen, which can increase the osteogenic potential. Surgical access to the donor bone is easily obtained through the incision, extending distally to the last molar. Portions of donor bone can be removed with curettes, as they are similar in thickness to eggshells, and partial regeneration of the tuberosity can occur afterwards.[14]

Histologically, there are three different processes associated with the success of bone grafts: osteogenesis, osteoinduction and osteoconduction. Studies show that cancellous bone grafts resorb less than cortical bone grafts, and the fact that they are more permeable to vascularization contributes to secondary stability and complete recovery. Cortical bone has the advantage of helping to anchor the implant because it has a higher density of inorganic matrix, allowing for primary stability. Therefore, based on the potential for primary stability and vascular permeability, the best results with autogenous grafts are obtained when using mono-cortical grafts containing cancellous bone and cortical bone in the same bone block, taking care to ensure that the cancellous portion is positioned in contact with the recipient bed.[13]

Significant resorption of the autogenous graft has been observed after the first 6 months of repair, except in the presence of loading or stimulation, which is an extremely relevant factor for the installation of implants at the same time as maxillary sinus elevation. Thus, the immediate installation of implants with maxillary sinus grafting is strongly related to a reduction in bone resorption.[14] In this context, previous studies have shown the presence of bone tissue around implants after 5 to 10 years, 90% of which had bone tissue covering the apex of the implant.[15] However, other authors have reported resorption rates of around 40% for autogenous bone, indicating that it should be associated with bovine bone in order to delay resorption of the material used to fill the sinus cavity.[14,]

### 2.3.2 Allografts or homogenous grafts

Homogenous bone grafts are classified as being of homogenous origin when the donated bone comes from individuals of the same species, but who are genetically different. The use of homogenous bone grafts from bone banks has aroused a lot of interest among surgeons, as they offer advantages such as reduced surgical time, lower morbidity, reduced vascular-nerve damage and infections. When large amounts of bone tissue are required, with consequent difficulty in obtaining an autogenous graft of satisfactory dimensions, especially in patients of advanced age and systemic impairment, the most assertive indication is the use of bone grafts from bone banks .[17]

Bone grafts have been used to increase the process of bone regeneration. Homogenous bone grafts from bone banks have emerged as an alternative in reconstructive surgery, as they have advantages such as their osteoinductive potential, storability, availability, mechanical resistance and eliminate the need for a donor site from the patient himself. Paraendodontic surgery, periodontal regeneration, orthognathic surgery, maxillary sinus lift and reconstruction of atrophic alveolar ridge are some of the indications for the use of homologous bone grafts in dentistry .[18]

The use of homologous material from bone banks is proving to be a very useful tool for dentistry, with the aim of regenerating lost bone tissue in the jaws. However, access to this type of material is difficult due to the low supply of bone banks in Brazilian hospitals that are qualified and structured for tissue preparation and storage.[17]

### 2.3.3 Heterogeneous xenografts or grafts

Given the difficulties involved in obtaining bone grafts from autogenous sources, bone substitutes from bovine species have been preferred by dental professionals due to their relative ease of sterilization and storage.[18]

The various biomaterials available for maxillary sinus augmentation have different biological behaviors depending on their origin, shape, size, porosity and rate of degradation. These differences directly affect the rate and time of bone formation. Bio-Oss® is a deprotected, slowly resorbed bovine xenograft, chemically and physically identical to human bone, in the form of cortical granules, with 75% to 80% porosity and a vast network of interconnected macro and micro pores, which facilitates angiogenesis and the migration of osteoblasts. Research has reaffirmed that the brief presence of Bio-Oss® incorporated into cancellous bone creates a dense network by reinforcing the mass of bone tissue and improving its ability to withstand the load forces transmitted by dental implants.[5]

### 2.3.4 Alloplastics

Alloplastics are bioinert and bioactive materials of synthetic origin that can be porous, crystalline, amorphous or granular, which should favor the formation of stable bonds with the newly formed bone, their functionality is through the formation of a framework for angiogenesis and consequently bone neoformation.[6]

In 1996, hydroxyapatite ($Ca_{10}(Po_4)_6(OH)_2$) was identified as one of the most effective osteoconductive biomaterials, consisting of a calcium phosphate salt which can be resorbable or non-resorbable. Hydroxyapatite (HA) particles are rendered non-resorbable by undergoing a synthesis process in which they are heat-treated at up to 1100 degrees Celsius, transforming the particles into a super-dense, compact and insoluble material that is suitable for filling large bone losses. Resorbable hydroxyapatite is indicated when the purpose of the material is bone replacement. As it is not synthesized, it resorbs slowly over 4 to 6 months and the fact that it is an inorganic material does not induce an antigenic reaction.[18]

Biphasic ceramics are alloplastic biomaterials made up of hydroxyapatite and tricalcium phosphate (TCP). They can be porous or dense and have osteoconductive properties by establishing a macro-structure for bone neoformation, which is a biomaterial that has a certain similarity to mineral bone. HA and β-TCP ceramics, on the other hand, are resorbed in a shorter period of time and have osteoconductive and osteoinductive properties due to the higher concentration of TCP, which increases the presence of micro pores, a fundamental characteristic that osteoinductive materials must have in order for osteogenitor cells to penetrate and find a good framework for bone neoformation.[20]

## 2.4 Performance of grafting biomaterials used in maxillary sinus lift surgery.

Costa, Trevisan Jûnior[21] (2007) report a clinical case in which a homologous bone graft was used from the bone bank of the Hospital das Clinicas in Curitiba, showing the use of this type of bone graft as an alternative in cases of atrophy in the posterior region of the maxilla, thus offering a lower degree of morbidity to patients during and after surgery. After surgery, biopsies were taken which showed osteogenesis in the area receiving the homogenous graft.

Stacchi[22] (2008) carried out a study using fresh-frozen homologous bone for maxillary sinus augmentation in ten individuals and found, five months after the grafting, by means of biopsy and histomorphometric evaluation under light microscopy, that the majority of the specimens showed neoformed bone completely integrated with the pre-existing bone. It was concluded that fresh-frozen homologous bone is a biocompatible material that can be successfully used in the reconstruction of maxillary sinuses without interfering with the bone repair process.

Contar et al.[23] (2009) demonstrated that fresh-frozen bone can be a successful graft material for the treatment of maxillary defects; appropriate surgical techniques allow this bone to be used safely in regions that will be implanted, making it a suitable alternative to autogenous grafts. Lately, the most commonly used allogeneic graft is lyophilized bone, the advantage of which is that there is no need to perform a second surgery at another site; its main disadvantage is that there is no phase I of osteogenesis.

Trindade-Suedam[24] et al. (2010) in a study of twenty rabbits that underwent maxillary sinus lift surgery with autogenous graft, bioglass, autogenous graft associated with platelet-rich plasma (PRP); and bioglass associated with platelet-rich plasma concluded that the best graft is still autogenous graft and the association with platelet-rich plasma shows no significant differences.

Lee et al.[25] (2012) evaluated the histomorphometric and clinical results of maxillary sinus floor elevation using deproteinized bovine biomaterial. Maxillary sinuses with a residual vertical height of <5 mm were grafted with the bovine biomaterial nine months before implant placement. At the time of implant surgery, some bone samples from patients were taken and subjected to histological and histomorphometric analysis. The percentages of regenerated bone and residual graft material were 19% and 40%, respectively. The implants placed in neoformed bone had a survival rate of 100% after a mean follow-up of 3 years. The average vertical height obtained was 7.9 mm. The use of bovine biomaterial to elevate the maxillary sinus floor is a predictable method for gaining vertical bone height in the posterior maxilla.

Lindgren et al.[26] (2012) compared bifacial calcium phosphate grafting with inorganic bovine bone grafting for maxillary sinus floor augmentation in the same patient. Partially or totally edentulous patients who required bilateral sinus augmentation were included in the study. Eight months after grafting, the dental implants were placed. After three years of graft healing, biopsy samples were obtained from the grafted areas for histological and histomorphometric analysis. After 3 years, a similar amount of newly formed bone was present, regardless of the biomaterial used. The choice of biomaterial does not seem to influence implant survival rates.

Oliveira et al.[27] (2012) carried out a study in dog alveoli with biomaterials associated or not with platelet-rich plasma and observed a more advanced repair in alveoli with PRP compared to alveoli without PRP.

Cardoso[7] (2013) carried out a study to evaluate the osteoconductive behavior of three different biomaterials, Osteoscaf (BoneTec Corp TRT Toronto Canada), BIO-Oss (Geistlich Biomaterials, wolhusen, CH Switzerland) and BoneCeramic (Straumann Institute AG Basel Switzerland) and to compare them with the osteoinductive behavior of autogenous cortico-medullary bone from the iliac crest. For this study, 66 male rabbits underwent grafting procedures. A total of 132 maxillary sinuses were organized into 4 groups according to the grafting material applied, with 11 sinuses in each group. The performance of the grafts was evaluated at intervals of 2-48 weeks after surgery using cone beam tomography, micro-microscopic tomography and molecular analysis using the PCR technique. The results revealed that autogenous bone showed greater resorption over the period evaluated, while bone substitutes showed greater neoformation. Among the bone substitutes, Bio-Oss showed greater bone neoformation over time when compared to Osteoscaf and Boneceramic. The bone substitutes performed better than autogenous bone and Osteoscaf showed greater resorption among the groups in all periods.

Thiesen et al.[28] (2013) obtained satisfactory results when performing a maxillary sinus lift procedure using crushed autogenous bone obtained from the mandibular ramus. This was a female patient with a bone remnant of between 2 and 4 mm. The surgical technique chosen was access via the lateral window. After access, the sinus membrane was displaced

13 mm vertically and the implant was installed in the planned position. Autogenous bone particles were carefully placed around the implant, filling all the space created below the sinus membrane. After nine months, the patient returned to have the prosthesis made. At the end of the procedures, very favorable results were observed, demonstrated by the recovery of function as well as the patient's high level of satisfaction with the results obtained. It is therefore important to note that the results obtained are stable after 4 years of follow-up.

Machado[19] (2014) carried out a clinical study involving 13 patients with pneumatized maxillary sinuses and the need for posterior dental rehabilitation. A total of 26 maxillary sinuses were submitted to the grafting procedure with maxillary sinus elevation. The purpose of the study was to volumetrically evaluate the bifacial porous ceramic graft (GenPhos-Porosa) in the proportion of 70% HA and 30% $\beta$-TCP compared to autogenous graft after 4 months of surgery. All patients underwent the grafting procedure where one sinus was filled with the ceramic biomaterial and the other with autogenous bone removed from the ramus or chin. Four months later, volume loss and bone remodeling were measured by computerized tomography. The percentage of maintenance of the grafted volume was higher for GenPhos with only 9% loss after 4 months, while autogenous bone had 44%. This fact leads to the conclusion that GenPhos is a promising and predictable material in terms of maintenance of the grafted volume for subsequent installation of implants in the maxillary sinus region.

Moraes et al.[15] (2015) performed a grafting procedure on a patient who had extensive pneumatization of the maxillary sinus for the subsequent installation of implants, the case was performed using the lateral window opening access technique and the deposition of HA-based biomaterial associated with cell-rich plasma with the addition of anticoagulants. The association of HA with cell-rich plasma aims to use growth factors to accelerate healing. After a period of 6 months, bone neoformation and the ability to install implants were observed on the grafted area. Bone residues from the instrumentation process were used for anatomopathological analysis, where it was possible to observe bone fragments with irregular and fragmented trabeculae, made up of osteocytes with typical nuclei and a matrix with irregular areas of calcification. Presence of osteoblasts absence of osteoclasts stretches of dense fibrous proliferation consisting of typical nucleus fibroblasts involving amorphous material also leading to the conclusion that the material used for bone grafting in maxillary sinus floor elevation surgery proved to be an effective alternative.

Ponte[29] (2016) carried out a systematic literature review of the variety of grafts available for maxillary sinus lifts in order to compare the use of *Bio-Oss®* with autogenous bone in terms of implant survival rates. Clinical-comparative articles on the use of *Bio-Oss®* and autogenous bone for maxillary sinus lifts in PubMed, Embase and the Cochrane Library were searched for, resulting in a total of 709 articles which, after the exclusion of duplicates, were reduced to 672 which had their abstracts read and within the established criteria only 60 articles were selected for full reading and among these only 8 allowed a fair comparative analysis because they presented methodological similarities. When the evaluation criterion was implant survival rate in the grafted area, the highest success rate in cases where only *Bio-Oss®* or associated with autogenous bone was used was 100%, while in cases where the graft was composed solely of autogenous bone, the highest rate was 82.4%. The number of randomized clinical trials on the subject is still scarce, preventing a meta-analysis from being carried out. However, it was possible to conclude that when using autogenous bone alone, *Bio-Oss®* alone or both options concomitantly, good results were achieved in terms of implant survival rates. These rates were similarly high and there was no statistically significant difference between the materials. Given the results found, it is not possible to establish BioOss® as the gold standard for maxillary sinus lift procedures, but we can use it as safely as we use autogenous bone, which is still the current gold standard.

| Grafting material | Advantages | Disadvantages |
| --- | --- | --- |
| Autogenous bone | The gold standard of grafting materials because it has OSteoInductive, Osteoconductive and OSteogenic potential, contains live Immunocompatible cells and is easily obtained ' .[1113] | Removal of the donor site is limited, requiring additional surgical intervention, generating morbidity and the need for longer recovery times, and the risk of major graft volume loss during the repair period ' .[1214] |
| Homogeneous Allograft | It eliminates the need for surgical removal and consequently eliminates the risk of vasculonervous lesions and infections at the donor site. It can be used in large quantities, has mechanical strength and osteoinductive and osteoconductive potential .[17] | Difficult to obtain due to the preparation and storage process, which is not very accessible; has a high resorption rate; has antigenic potential and does not promote an osteogenic reaction; has a high cost .[17] |
| Heterogeneous Xenograft | It has the same advantages as homogenous grafts and is characterized by a reduction in antigenic potential, accessibility, storage capacity and costs. (Bio-Oss) and maintenance of the grafted volume[7] - .[29] | No osteogenic action and low cost .[729] |
| Alloplastics | No need for a donor surgical site; available in large quantities; osteoconductive capacity, maintenance of grafted volume (HA)®-[18] | Risk of rejection followed by infection, slower replacement with bone tissue, low mechanical strength[1] ®. |

**Figure-1 Main characteristics that influence the choice of grafting material to be used in maxillary sinus**

lift procedures.

Based on the different origins of the grafting materials used for maxillary sinus elevation, regardless of the surgical technique, figure-1 was drawn up in order to make a comparative analysis of osteogenic capacity, which is still only possible for autogenous bone, but osteoinductive and osteoconductive potential is present in the various biomaterials of different origins. The advantage of eliminating the need for a donated surgical site is common to the various biomaterials and although each material has peculiar characteristics in terms of origin and composition, both are eligible for the grafting procedure although they induce different levels of results.

## 3 Conclusion

By studying different types of grafting materials, it was possible to note that qualifying the success of grafted biomaterials is quite complex. From a clinical point of view, there is a tendency to attribute success to the graft based on the simple presence of mineralized material with a firm consistency and the ability to retain the implant. However, real success is based on histological analysis of the grafted region, where it is possible to see more details about the bone replacement process and to qualify the newly formed tissue, which has a great influence on the longevity of clinical success.

Although autogenous bone grafting is still considered the gold standard, the characteristics of *Bio-Oss®* bovine xenografts (Geistlich Biomaterials, Wolhusen, CH, Switzerland) have shown satisfactory histological results in terms of bone replacement, These advantages make its use more attractive, leading professionals to select this type of graft as the material of first choice in maxillary sinus floor elevation surgeries.

## 4-References†


1. Colussi CF, Patel FS. Use and Need for Prosthodontics in Brazil: advances, perspectives and challenges. Sau. & Transf. Soc. 2016; 7(1):41-48.

2. Silva BCS, Carvalho PSP, Vedovato E, Bassi APF, Conforte JJ, Ponzoni D. Retrospective study of the survival rate of implants installed by professionals with different degrees of experience in implant dentistry. RFO, Passo Fundo. 2015; 20(3):295-301.

3. Reis JC, Calixto RFE. Review article Maxillary sinus lift surgery enabling the use of implants. Investigaçâo Saùde.2015;14(1):164- 68.


---

† According to FACIT's Course Conclusion Work norms, based on Vancouver standards. Available at: http://www.nlm.nih.gov/bsd/uniform_requirements.html.

4.     Bucco Junior RLS, Silva TPT, Miranda CCL, Koelsch MHD, Rosa AJB. Bilateral maxillary sinus elevation using 100 percent alloplastic biomaterial for posterior rehabilitation of an atrophic maxilla. Dent. press implantol. 2015; 9(1):42-56.

5.     Albuquerque AFM,,Cardoso IML, Silva JSPS, Germano, Dantas WRM, Gondim ALMF. Maxillary sinus lift using freeze-dried bone associated with immediate installation of a Morse cone implant: case report. RFO, Passo Fundo. 2014; 19(1):129-34.

6.     Dantas TS, Lelisa ER, Navesb LZ, Fernandes-Netoa AJ, Magalhaesa D. Bone Graft Materials and their Applications in Dentistry. UNOPAR Cient Ciênc Biol Saùde 2011;13(2):131 -5.

7.     Cardoso CL. Analysis of the use of Osteoscaf as a bone substitute in maxillary sinus lift surgery. [Doctoral dissertation] Bauru: Bauru School of Dentistry University of Sao Paulo;2013.

8.     Mazaro JVQ, Pellizzer EP, Santiago Junior JF, Verril FR, Melo CC. Longitudinal evaluation of two sinus lift techniques. Rev. Cir. Traumatol. Buco-Maxilo- Fac. Camaragibe. 2013; 3(3):09-16.

9.     Salomao M, Siqueira JTT. Guided bone regeneration through a barrier exposed to the oral environment after exodontia. Case report. Rev. Bras. Implant. 2010; 16(3):5-7.

10.    Ferreira RMD, Dias ECLCLM, Harari ND, Cardoso ES, Vidigal Junior GM. Is there an association between the angle formed by the lower third of the medial and lateral walls of the maxillary sinus and the risk of membrane perforation? A cross-sectional study. ImplantNews. 2014; 11(6):148-152.

11.    Vicente JC, Hernandez-Vallejo G, Brana-Abascal P, Pena I. Maxillary sinus augmentation with autologous bone harvested from the lateral maxillary wall combined with bovine-derived hydroxyapatite: clinical and histologic observations. Clin Oral Implants Res. 2010;21(4):430-8.

12.    Stricker A, Voss PJ, Gutwald R, Schramm A, Schmelzeisen R. Maxillary sinus floor augmentation with autogenous bone grafts to enable placement of SLA-surfaced implants: preliminary results after 15-40 months. Clin Oral Implants Res. 2003; 14:207-12.

13.    Milhomem MLA. Intraoral autogenous grafts in implant dentistry: Literature review. Revista Amazônia Science & Health. 2014;2(3):32-37.

14.    Sbordone, L., Levin, L., Guidetti, F., Sbordone, C., Glikman, A., & Schwartz- Arad, D. Apical and marginal bone alterations around implants in maxillary sinus augmentation

grafted with autogenous bone or bovine bone material and simultaneous or delayed dental implant positioning. Clinical oral implants research. 2011; 22(5):485-491.

15.   Moraes CW, Guerrieri LL, Petrilli G,Nantes LRR, Costa-Frutuoso JR. Maxillary sinus floor elevation surgery with alloplastic graft associated with platelet-rich plasma: case report. 2015; Rev. Ibirapuera. 2 (10):17-26

16.   Mathias MVR, Bassanta AD, Ramalho AS, Saba-Chujfi E, Simone JL. Autogenous graft with donor sites in the oral cavity. RGO (Porto Alegre). 2003 Oct; 51(4): 249-56.

17.   Souza DO, Almeida Jr E, Barreto IC, Oliveira TFL, Araùjo RPC. Applications of bone bank grafts in dentistry. R. Ci. med. biol. 2010; 9(1):45-48.

18.   Camargo CD, Branco MV, Hoppe EF. Five-year follow-up of maxillary reconstruction with fresh-frozen homogenous grafts. ImplantNews. 2010;7(2):189-193.

19.   Machado RQP. Volumetric evaluation of a bilateral maxillary sinus lift procedure using a porous bifacial ceramic: randomized clinical study with evaluation after four months of healing. [Master's dissertation] Bauru: Bauru School of Dentistry University of São Paulo;2014.

20.   Oliveira LSAF,      Conceiçâo Silva Oliveira, Machado APL, Rosa FP.

Biomaterials with application in bone regeneration - method of analysis and future perspectives. R. Ci. med. biol. 2010; 9(1):37-44.

21.   Costa RR, Trevisan Jùnior W. Bilateral maxillary sinus lift using homogenous bone from a bone bank: a viable alternative. ImplantNews.2007;4(5)513-520, 2007.

22.   Stacchi C, Orsini G, Di Iorio, D, Breschi L, & Di Lenarda, R.Clinical, Histologic, and Histomorphometric Analyses of Regenerated Bone in Maxillary Sinus Augmentation Using Fresh Frozen Humam Bone Allografts. J. Periodontol. 2008; (79):1789-1796.

23.   Contar CMM, Sarot JR, Bordini J, Galvâo GH, Nicolau GV, Machado MAN. Maxillary Ridge Augmentation With Fresh-Frozen Bone Allografts. J. Oral Maxillofac Surg, 2009. v.67, p.1280-1285.

24.   Trindade-Suedam IK, Morais J, Faeda RS, Leite FR.M Tosoni GM, Neto CB, Marcantonio JR. Bioglass Associated With Leukocyte-Poor Platelet-Rich Plasma in the Rabbit Maxillary Sinus: Histomorphometric, Densitometric, and Fractal Analysis. Journal and Oral Implantology. 2010; 36(5):333-343.

25. Lee D.Z., Chen S.T., Darby I.B. Maxillary sinus floor elevation and grafting with deproteinized bovine bone mineral: a clinical and histomorphometric study. Clin Oral

Implants Res. 2012. 23 (8):918-24.

26.   Lindgren C., Mordenfeld A., Johansson C.B., Hallman M. A 3-year clinical follow-up of implants placed in two different biomaterials used for sinus augmentation. Int Journal Oral Maxillofac Implantes. 2012; 27 (5) :1151-62.

27.   Oliveira B, Camarini C, Salavar M, Pavan A, Camarini ET. The use of equine (Bio-gen) and bovine (Genox) bone associated or not with PRP in mandibular dog sockets: split-mouth design with histological analysis. Implant News. 2012;9(6)195-269.

28.   Thinsen MJ, Azzolin AC, Orellana AP, Souza JR Vieira RA, Padovan LEM, Claudino M. Maxillary sinus lift with autogenous graft and immediate implant installation: four-year follow-up. Salusvita Bauru. 2013: 32(1):87-102.

29.   Ponte ME. Implant survival after maxillary sinus lift using autogenous bone graft, *bio-oss®* or a combination of autogenous bone and *bio-oss®*. Systematic literature review. [Master's dissertation] Porto Alegre: School of Dentistry, Pontifical Catholic University of Rio Grande do Sul; 2016.

# CHAPTER III. TRANSOPERATIVE AND POSTOPERATIVE COMPLICATIONS IN REHABILITATION WITH OSSEOINTEGRATED DENTAL IMPLANTS: THE MAIN COMPLICATIONS AND THERAPEUTIC SOLUTIONS

Janderson Castro dos Santos1 Rodrigo Dalla Lana Mattiello2

1- Graduated in Dentistry ITPAC Araguaína-TO, Specialist in Implant Dentistry FACIT Araguaína-TO, Master in Dentistry São Leopoldo Mandic Campinas-SP. 2- Graduated in Dentistry and specialist in Implant Dentistry at the Federal University of Mato Grosso do Sul Campo Grande MS, Master in Health and Development at the Federal University of Mato Grosso do Sul Campo Grande MS, PhD student in Implant Dentistry at São Leopoldo Mandic Campinas SP, Coordinator of the specialization course in implant dentistry at the Faculty of Sciences of Tocantins FACIT Araguaína TO.

## Summary

The high rate of tooth loss, improved life expectancy and financial viability have increased the search for oral rehabilitation with osseointegrated implants. Although rehabilitation with implants is a safe method with high success rates, as it is a surgical procedure involving interdisciplinary knowledge in the areas of oral surgery, occlusion and prosthetics, performed in an environment with difficult access and restricted visibility, complications can occur. The aim of this non-systematic review was to carry out a bibliographic survey to describe the main trans-operative and post-operative surgical complications related to implant dentistry, as well as to report on the main preventative measures and the fundamental solutions for repairing or limiting damage. The results showed that post-operative complications are the most frequently reported in the literature and can be of traumatic origin resulting from failures committed during surgery or of infectious origin.

The occurrence of major intra- and post-operative complications was generally more frequent in cases where grafting procedures were associated with implant installation. As for complications of trans-operative origin, these were classified as occasional accidents or iatrogenic injury to anatomical structures, with complications of this class being less frequently reported. It should be emphasized that knowing the main occurrences and causes of intra- and post-operative complications is of great value so that preventive measures can be taken or repair actions can be taken immediately in order to limit further injury to implant dentistry patients.

**Keywords**: dental implants; osseointegration; transoperative complications, postoperative complications.

1-Introduction

Implant dentistry is a leading specialty in dentistry and offers the best treatment options for the oral rehabilitation of partially or totally edentulous patients. Due to its high success rates, implant dentistry has proven to be highly predictable and safe, offering the best advantages over other methods of oral rehabilitation (Silva et al.[1] 2015).

The main advantage of implants is that they are a fixed prosthesis with an excellent degree of stability, providing chewing safety thanks to the phenomenon of osseointegration, which is the process of direct structural and functional connection between living bone and the surface of an implant subjected to occlusal loads. (Silva et al.[1] 2015) report that osseointegration has predictable, reproducible and stable results over time, and the success rate is between 96.99% and 97.15% over a five-year follow-up.

The high rate of dental loss has led to a growing search for methods of oral rehabilitation, which has increased the incidence of patients being rehabilitated with osseointegrated implants. Even though this is a safe method with high levels of success, indiscriminate indication and a lack of technical and surgical planning can lead to failure and compromise the final result of the treatment.

With the increase in the number of implants installed, there has also been an increase in the occurrence of implant complications reported in the literature. According to a survey on current issues in dentistry in 2000, published by the American Dental Association (ADA), it was observed that over a four-year period (1995-1999) the average number of implants placed by dentists each year rose from 37.7 to 56.2. Among the dentists who took part in the survey, a high number of general practitioners practiced implant dentistry in their daily routine, showing that this method of rehabilitation has become more popular.

Technological advances, improvements in the population's quality of life, cost reductions and the increase in the number of dental professionals are factors that have facilitated access to oral rehabilitation using implants, and as more patients are rehabilitated with implants, the number of complications involving the specialty also increases .[3]

Although implant dentistry procedures are safe and have high success rates, it is important to note that it is a complex therapy involving surgical intervention, requiring adequate patient health conditions, professional skills and scientific technical knowledge that are essential to minimize operative complications and the expected injuries are properly controlled. Complications are unforeseen complications in the treatment and when not resolved in a timely manner can lead to treatment failure.

Knowing which are the most frequent intercurrences in the day-to-day life of the implant dentistry clinic, as well as adopting measures to prevent and control possible damage, is invaluable information so that the professional can act correctly when faced with such a situation. Therefore, the aim of this study is to carry out a bibliographical survey to describe the main trans-operative and post-operative surgical complications related to rehabilitation with osseointegrated implants, to report on the main preventive measures, and to set out the fundamental solutions for repairing or limiting the damage caused.

**2-Review of the Literature**

**2.1- The teaching of implantology in Brazil**

Dentistry in general is a profession that requires a lot of dedication to study in order to acquire a good theoretical basis that becomes effective in guiding clinical practice and, as a result, operative technique skills are achieved. In order to find out and compare how implant dentistry is taught in undergraduate courses in different regions of Brazil, Ferreira [4] (2014) evaluated 52 teaching institutions and the result was that the subject of implant dentistry is offered in 26. 9% of the institutions in the fourth quarter,9% of the institutions in the fourth year of the undergraduate course, 34.6% of the colleges reported that the teaching staff of the subject is made up of 2 teachers, and the format of the classes in 83.3% of the institutions are theoretical and laboratory, 6.7% theoretical, laboratory and clinical. It is also important to note that 2.5% of the institutions do not offer implant dentistry as a subject, 64.2% offer it as an option and in 33.3% of the faculties it is a compulsory subject.

The surgeon's skill and experience are important factors in the success of dental implants. Andesson et al.[5] (1995) reported that general dentists with 8 days of training obtained similar clinical results for the placement of single implants compared to the results obtained in a specialty clinic. On the other hand, Zoghbi et al.[6] (2011) reported that the surgeon's experience has a positive influence on the osseointegration of dental implants. Surgical experience was defined based on the number of implants placed: less experienced professionals had placed less than 50 dental implants; more experienced professionals had placed more than 50. The results showed that more experienced professionals achieved a higher rate of osseointegration (94.4%) than less experienced professionals (84.0%). Lambert et al.[7] (1997) reported that implant failure rates were lower when implants were placed by an experienced surgeon. Al-Sabbagh, Bhavsar[8] (2015) reinforce these statements by reporting that specialists in implant dentistry have a better critical sense when developing solutions for each case treated, enabling them to acquire better experience and consequently better treatment success rates.

## 2.2- Historical Context of Implant Dentistry

Since the beginning of the 20th century, various authors have proposed different techniques and materials for oral rehabilitation using dental implants, but it wasn't until 1952 when physiologist Per-Ingvar Branemark discovered by chance the intimate relationship between the surface of titanium and bone tissue, proving the phenomenon of osseointegration, which was the first major step towards the foundation of implant dentistry. A few years later, Branemark himself defined the process of osseointegration as: a direct structural and functional connection between viable normal bone tissue and the functioning implant.

In 1988, during a conference held in Washington, D.C., the general criteria that determine the success of implants were established:

> The individual implant must remain immobile when tested clinically.

> When examined on radiographs, radiolucent evidence in the peri-implant region should be absent.

> The average vertical bone loss should be less than 0.02 mm per year after the first year.

> Absence of persistent pain, discomfort or infection attributable to the implant.

> The design of the implant should not prevent the prosthesis or crown from being placed with a satisfactory appearance for the patient and the dentist.

The clinical and radiographic features that characterize the success of implant installation remain the same as those proposed in 1988. However, during the surgical stage of implant installation, some complications can occur and interfere with the final result of the rehabilitation process[9] . In the course of this article, the main intra- and post-operative complications arising from the installation of dental implants will be presented.

## 2.3- Classifications of operative complications and the main occurrences recorded in the literature.

Nòia et al.[10] (2010) classified surgical complications in implantology according to the time of implant installation as follows:

•	**Transoperative complications** - These occur during the surgical procedure. The main **complications** in this category are bone fenestrations, injury to the inferior alveolar nerve and implant positioning errors.

- **Post-operative complications** - These are the problems that occur after implant installation surgery, among which gingival tissue dehiscence, surgical site infection and paresthesia of the inferior alveolar nerve are the most frequently mentioned.

When comparing the level of incidence between trans-operative and post-operative accidents, there was a higher frequency of post-operative accidents, 9.75% compared to 3.60%, according to a study carried out when 532 medical records were evaluated based on standardized criteria developed in the department of oral and maxillofacial surgery at FOP/Unicamp Piracicaba-SP. Of the 532 patients treated, 19 had some kind of complication recorded, the most frequent being bone fenestration as a trans-operative complication and surgical site infection in the case of post-operative problems (Noia et al.[10] 2010).

Silva et al.[11] (2010) carried out a retrospective study analyzing 660 records of patients treated at the Oral and Maxillofacial Surgery Department of the Piracicaba School of Dentistry - Unicamp over a period of 8 years. The medical records were rigorously evaluated and surgical complications and complications were quantified and classified according to their occurrence. Among the 660 patients in this study, 18.03% had some kind of complication when the procedure did not involve any alveolar reconstruction technique, while in cases where the implants were associated with alveolar reconstruction, the rate of complications was 36.16%. The main occurrences quantified in descending order in implant surgeries without associated grafting were: Bone fenestrations, Perforation of the maxillary sinus membrane, Insufficient bone height, Bleeding, Injury to the inferior alveolar nerve and Lack of primary implant stability. When analyzing the possible factors that contributed to surgical complications, it was noted that patients who underwent surgery with planning using only panoramic radiography were twice as likely to make a mistake, while patients who underwent alveolar reconstruction procedures were up to four times more likely to have complications than those who did not need such a procedure.

Bjarni et al.[12] (2014) conducted a systematic review of the literature to estimate and compare the survival rate and complications of esthetic, biological and technical origin of implant-supported prostheses. For this study, articles on the subject published before and after the year 2000 were included, including randomized controlled clinical studies, controlled clinical studies, prospective studies, retrospective and prospective case studies. A total of 139 studies were selected according to the research criteria and these were divided into two groups, studies prior to the year 200 (n = 31) and a group of studies published after the year 2000 (n = 108) and then the survival rate and complications were calculated using a validated scientific instrument, and then the groups were compared according to the results.

It was observed that the 5-year survival rate of implant-supported dental prostheses was significantly increased in studies after the year 2000, from 93.5% to 97.1%. As for the occurrence of biological complications, the most commonly mentioned were perimplantitis, marginal bone loss, and signs of inflammation of different origins such as swelling, redness, and bleeding in soft tissues. The comparison between the occurrence of biological complications in articles published before 2000 showed that there was a reduction from 2.56% to 1.31% in the case of single implants, while in the case of multiple implants there was an increase from 1.54% to 1.97%.

## 2.4- Transoperative accidents and complications.

Implant dentistry, as an integral part of oral rehabilitation, is a major challenge in meeting the patient's needs, i.e. restoring function and aesthetics with all their implications: proper nutrition, phonetics, aesthetic beauty, emotional health, self-esteem, social acceptance, and like any surgical and/or clinical procedure, implant dentistry is also subject to failures, which increases the professional's responsibility to take certain precautions and pay attention to some fundamental points in order to eliminate or at least minimize the occurrence and severity of these failures and complications.

Ramalho-Ferreira et al.[13] (2010) reported the most likely transoperative complications and classified the occurrences directly related to the implant and its structure: Unfavorable position and angulation, swallowing or aspiration of instruments and/or implant components, and violation of anatomical structures such as: Inferior Alveolar Nerve Injury, iatrogenic bleeding, intra-sinusal implant insertion, mandibular fracture, iatrogenic bleeding. These complications will be discussed in the following topics, addressing the reasons why they may occur, as well as measures to prevent and control any damage caused.

## 2.4.1- Swallowing or aspirating instruments and/or implant components

During surgery, patients are often kept in the supine or semi-recumbent position while small instruments are taken into the oral cavity, which is a dark, restricted environment where the humidity of saliva in contact with the instruments and gloves increases the risk of accidental swallowing or aspiration of instruments or parts of the implant. When implants are inserted into the surgical socket, one of the concerns is that the implant's capture key escapes and it falls into the oral cavity because, as well as being contaminated by contact with saliva, it can be swallowed or aspirated.

In cases where patients are sedated, the risk is higher, as their cough reflexes will be reduced. In the case of swallowing, if the object does not have a sharp point, it can travel through the gastrointestinal tract and be eliminated; even so, a chest X-ray should be taken to make sure that it is not an asymptomatic aspiration. If the object is small and is aspirated, partially obstructing the airways, the patient should be immediately taken to an emergency center, receiving supplementary oxygen during the transfer, where they should undergo a laryngoscopy or bronchoscopy, which should be performed as soon as possible to remove the object. In implantology, the instrument most often involved in these accidents is the digital key used to place the *cover* or implant at the end of surgery or during the reopening phase .[14]

This type of accident can be prevented by the following procedures: using gauze to block access to the oropharynx, attaching dental floss to the small devices used in dental care, positioning the dental chair upright, working with experienced assistants, using suckers .[14]

## 2.4.2- Violation of anatomical structures

The availability of 3 to 5 mm of bone after the root apex of the teeth adjacent to the implant bed is necessary for primary stability, and is useful for avoiding the violation of anatomical structures such as the nasal fossa, the incisive canal in the anterior maxillary region, the maxillary sinus in the posterior maxillary region, as well as the inferior alveolar nerve and the mental foramen in mandibular interventions. The vertical elevation of the sinus with an osteotome and the placement of a wide-neck implant reduce the likelihood of an immediate implant being inserted into the maxillary sinus cavity[15] . Obtaining cross-sectional radiographic images to locate the maxillary sinus, nasal cavity, inferior alveolar nerve and lingual nerve is useful to avoid violating this anatomical structure where it is recommended to preserve a minimum of 2 mm free space between the apex of the implant and the surrounding structures; the use of depth limiting devices is also an alternative to be used as a preventive measure .[16]

## 2.4.3- Inferior Alveolar Nerve Injury

The selection of implants of inadequate length, failures to measure the vertical extension in the preparation of the surgical socket are the most likely errors related to trauma, which can cause compression or even rupture of the Inferior Alveolar Nerve. In cases where after implant installation the patient reports symptoms of paresthesia in the lower lip and if this persists for more than a week, a CT scan should be requested to determine a possible causal relationship with the implant. If this is confirmed, removal should be preceded.

These nerve injuries can be treated with laser therapy, medication and microsurgery, and early removal of the implant is considered a key factor for a better prognosis of this damage.

It is important that these measures are started as soon as possible after the surgeon-dentist realizes that nerve damage has occurred .[17]

### 2.4.4- Mandibular fracture

As life expectancy increases, more and more elderly people with total edentulism and severe bone resorption are coming to the implant dentistry clinic in search of rehabilitation solutions. Care for these patients must be rigorously planned in order to avoid surgical complications such as mandibular bone fractures, which usually result from untimely maneuvers and very traumatic surgical manipulation. When a mandibular fracture occurs, the patient usually presents with pain and swelling on palpation of the alveolar ridge. When the fracture does not present with mobility on palpation, treatment can be carried out by reducing the mandibular masticatory forces, which includes liquid/pasty feeding and removing the use of prostheses for a period of 4 to 6 weeks. Deviated and unstable fractures require surgical reduction and rigid internal fixation with plates and screws or titanium mesh adapted to the base of the mandible .[18]

### 2.4.5- Iatrogenic bleeding

Usually caused when the lingual cortical bone of the mandible is perforated during the milling or implant installation procedure, causing injury to arteries in the floor of the mouth, branches of the lingual and facial arteries. Signs and symptoms appear with an increase in volume in the submandibular region and the floor of the mouth, causing the tongue to rise. In less serious cases, arterial ligation can be tried to stop the bleeding, but in more serious situations the patient should be transferred to a hospital .[19]

### 2.4.6- Intra-sinusal implant insertion

Inadvertent insertion of the implant into the maxillary sinus can occur both during the installation phase and during reopening or prosthetic manipulation of the implant. This is due to poor planning or inadequate surgical management, coupled with poor quality bone and low quantity, incorrect use of temporary mucosupported prostheses over the newly implanted area are also risk factors. The patient presents with a feeling of pressure in the face, diffuse headache and radiographically there is an increase in the radiopacity of the maxillary sinus. The implant should be removed via the Caldwell-Luc surgical approach, never via the insertion route, which causes destruction of the alveolar bone and is a very limited access route to the maxillary sinus. If the implant is not removed, it can cause acute or chronic sinusitis. Due to the anatomy and physiology of the posterior maxillary region, it is essential to ensure primary stability of the implant to prevent the risk of its displacement into the maxillary sinus. Prevention also comes from correct planning through imaging and care when inserting implants in the posterior maxilla .[20]

## 2.5- Main post-surgical complications

## 2.5.1- Infection

Post-operative infections in implantology occur in approximately 5% of cases, with varying degrees, ranging from moderate sinus infections, treated with antibiotics; others that develop oral fistulas; implant loss due to infection; total graft failure and maxillary sinusitis .[21,22]

Strict care must be taken to maintain the aseptic chain in implant surgery, as this is a dental procedure that can have major systemic repercussions when it involves the insertion of an intraosseous object, and even if the implant is biocompatible, the presence of microorganisms can interfere with bone physiology, leading to excessive inflammation and damaging the osseointegration process. In the daily routine of the dental practice, it is important to periodically monitor the sterilization cycles to make sure that the materials are being sterilized properly, and the surgical equipment must be made respecting the smallest details to protect the surgical field .[23]

Pre-medication with broad-spectrum antibiotics is recommended. Complete debridement of the infectious contents inside the alveoli after extraction and curettage of all granulation tissue are necessary. In cases of active diffuse infection, delayed implantation is recommended .[24]

## 2.5.2- -Bone overheating.

Bone is sensitive to temperature and overheating the bone during implant preparation can lead to necrosis of the bone tissue surrounding the dental implant. Less surgical trauma is expected when the procedure is carried out by skilled and experienced dentists, the skill of the operator being an important factor in the success of dental implants. Overheating of the bone should be avoided by the use of abundant irrigation and periodic replacement of drills to ensure cutting power, if bone drilling is carried out without adequate cooling, damage to the bone is increased because of heat generation[25] . A temperature higher than 47C° for 1 minute can cause irreversible damage to bone tissue; a temperature higher than 47C° can be reached within seconds during osteotomy preparation without irrigation.

The implant manufacturer's guidelines for drilling speed must be followed, low drill pressure on bone is also a determining factor in reducing the risk of trauma during drilling of dense bone .[26]

### 2.5.3- Surgical wound dehiscence

It is characterized by the opening of the surgical suture. Its main cause is excessive inflammation which results in the degradation of proteins in the extracellular matrix. He also notes that when extraction and implant installation take place in the same surgery, with no waiting time, the incidence of dehiscence is higher than if there was a wait of a few weeks between the procedures. Repeat sutures are also not recommended, as there is a tendency for a new rupture[10] . A recommended technique is to create small perforations in the exposed bone tissue, debridement of the necrotic tissue and abundant irrigation with saline solution so that the epithelium of the inserted gingiva can regenerate around the implant, forming a free gingival margin containing keratocytes on the surface. Studies have also shown that inducing superficial bleeding of the bone tissue stimulates cell migration and facilitates tissue regeneration .[27]

### 2.5.4- Surgical emphysema

Clinically, the patient has an increase in soft tissue volume due to the presence of subcutaneous air. When palpated, there is a cryptic appearance and pain, which can lead to obstructed breathing, cardiac function and retinal perfusion. Radiographically, the air inside the soft tissues appears as a radiolucent image. Its cause is associated with the introduction of air into the subcutaneous tissues or facial planes[28] . Subcutaneous emphysema in itself is innocuous and usually resolves without sequelae within a few days. However, the trapped air can migrate along the facial planes to deep structures, which can result in serious complications. The appearance of subcutaneous emphysema due to the use of a high-rotation pen is uncommon in dentistry, especially in implantology.

To avoid this, one option would be to use electric motors with straight and angled surgical tips. Correct diagnosis is essential in order to avoid further complications. They tend to regress spontaneously .[30]

### 2.5.5- Implant mobility

Implant mobility is a warning sign that the osseointegration process has failed. Clinically, the patient may feel pain when touching the implant. The causes are related to inadequate bone quality or inaccurate drilling for primary implant stability[31] . Treatment consists of removing the implant and replacing it with a larger one. In the case of minor mobility, there is the possibility of trying to extend the healing period to wait for osseointegration .[32]

### 2.5.6- Fenestration of the vestibular bone plate.

Among the complications related to the installation of immediate implants, fenestration and dehiscence have been reported as the most frequent among post-surgical complications[22] The most common areas for fenestration during the installation of immediate implants are the upper anterior teeth and premolars. To eliminate the risk of fenestration, a spherical drill positioned off-center towards the palatal side and along the alveolar ridge angulation should be performed to reduce the chances of fenestration of the buccal bone plate of the alveolar ridge. When these complications occur, bone regeneration may be possible; however, in some cases, delayed implant placement may be advisable.[13]

## 2.6- An overview of the most common complications described in the literature.

Oral rehabilitation using implants is a very safe procedure. Noia et al.[10] (2010) reported that in 532 patients, 86.65% of the cases treated did not have any trans-operative complications. Based on the bibliographic findings on the main trans-operative complications encountered in the preparation of this article, figure 1 was organized in order to classify the complications into injuries to anatomical structures and possible accidents.

As for post-operative complications, these are more frequent, around 36.74 % of implant-related surgical complications are post-operative and among these the most frequent are bone fenestrations followed by injuries to the inferior alveolar nerve and implant malposition[10] . Figure 2 below shows the post-operative complications mentioned in the literature and classifies them according to etiology, whether infectious or traumatic, as well as describing measures to prevent and control the damage caused.

| Transoperative complications | | Causes | Prevention Measures | What to do? |
|---|---|---|---|---|
| **Eventual Claim** | **Swallowing** instruments or implant components | Supine position of the patient in the reduced chair or cough reflexes during sedation. | | If non-sharp: elimination should be monitored through chest X-rays |
| | **Aspiration** of instruments or implant components | | Attention of operator and assistant, tying dental floss on small instruments, | Respiratory support should be provided and removal by laryngoscopy should be carried out (ENT specialist who should carry out the procedures). |
| **Injury to anatomical structures** | Injury to the inferior alveolar nerve | | Use a depth limiter | Removing the implant |
| | Invasion of the nasal fossa | | Watch out for vestibularization of the implant apex during installation | Removing the implant |

| Trans-operative complications | Prevention | What to do? |
|---|---|---|
| Maxillary sinus invasion | Failures in radiographic or tomographic planning / Perform sinus lift, or use depth limiters | Remove the implant and treat sinusitis with antibiotics |
| Mandibular fracture | Care with insertion torque and number of implants installed in the same region | If the fracture is stable: advise a reduction in chewing forces and a soft diet for 4 to 6 weeks. If the Fracture If the fracture is unstable: Rigid internal fixation with plates and screws should be carried out. |
| Bleeding | Perforation of the lingual bone wall of the mandible / Attention to lingual inclination of mandibular implants | Macerate the bleeding point, use bone wax or ligature the injured vessels. |

**Figure 1** - Distribution of the main trans-operative complications, prevention and management.

| | Post-operative complications | Prevention | 0 what to do? |
|---|---|---|---|
| **Surgical trauma** | Fenestration of the vestibular bone plate | When performing implant surgeries in areas with vestibular bone depressions or thin vestibular bone plates, it is important to have freeze-dried bone and collagen membrane available for immediate repair of the defect. | When traumatic, the gap should be filled with bone and covered with a collagen membrane. When it is of infectious origin, it usually leads to the loss of the implant. |
| | Bone overheating | Use new cutters with high cutting power and abundant irrigation | Monitor healing, which can lead to loss of the implant |
| | Emphysema | This is a very rare event and can be prevented by avoiding the use of pneumatic turbines in surgical procedures. | The important thing is to make sure that it's not an allergic crisis, because it returns spontaneously and gradually. |
| **Infections** | Surgical wound dehiscence | Maintenance of the aseptic chain and proper suturing, evaluation of the periodontal profile. | Control local inflammation and assess the inflammatory condition of the tissues to proceed with a new suture. |
| | Implant mobility | The occurrence of this event is closely associated with a breach of the aseptic chain or neglect of post-operative care. | Sign of inflammation and failure of osseointegration indicating need for implant removal |
| | Fistulas | | Generally, fistulas associated |

44

| | | with implants cause mobility and loss |
|---|---|---|
| Sinusitis | They are usually associated with trauma and can be prevented by precise radiographic planning. | Remove the causative factor and proceed with antibiotic therapy |

**Figure 2-** Post-operative complications, prevention measures and technical approaches to damage control.

## 3- CONCLUSION

•	Pre-operative planning and professional technical skill have been shown to reduce the risk of post-operative complications due to greater accuracy of experience in planning, indicating and applying surgical techniques and prosthetic solutions.

•	Pre-operative planning for implant dentistry involves knowledge of several areas, such as dental prosthetics, periodontics, occlusion, physiology, anatomy, radiology and pharmacology, since implant success is not restricted to osseointegration and maintenance;

•	Planning should focus on the possibility of achieving acceptable functional aesthetic rehabilitation that does not jeopardize the longitudinal nature of the case.

•	The frequency of trans-operative complications seems to be less frequent than post-operative complications, as there are few reports of such occurrences;

•	Trans- and post-operative complications are more frequent in cases of implants that involved a grafting procedure or immediate implants.

•	In the event of a trans-operative complication, knowing what to do immediately is fundamental to reducing any damage to the patient's integrity.

## 4-References‡


1.	Silva BCR, Paulo, Carvalho SP, Vedovato, E, Bassi, APF, Conforte JJ, D Ponzoni. D. Retrospective study of the survival rate of implants installed by professionals with different degrees of experience in implant dentistry. RFO, Passo Fundo 2015; 20 (3): 295-301.

2.	Frâncio L, Souza AM, Storrer CLM, Deliberador TM, Souza AC, Pizzatto E. et al. Treatment of periodontitis: literature review. Rev Sul-Bras Odontol. 2008; 6:75-81.

3.	Stuart JF. Complications in oral implantology: etiology, prevention and treatment. São


---


‡ In accordance with FACIT's Course Conclusion Work standards,　　based on Vancouver standards. Available at:
http://www.nlm.nih.gov/bsd/uniform_requirements.html.

Paulo Ed. Santos. Chap. 1 Implant complications: the scope of the problem. 2013. p.1-7.

4.      FERREIRA, J.P.R. Implant dentistry teaching in undergraduate course of dentistry, the case studies of an institution and the profile of the patients assisted at the clinic of Dental implantology of Faculdades de Odontogia - FAI. 2014. 74f. [Doctoral Thesis in Preventive and Social Dentistry] Araçatuba School of Dentistry, São Paulo State University, Araçatuba, 2014.

5.      Andersson B, Odman P, Lindvall AM, et al. Surgical and prosthodontic training of general practitioners for single tooth implants: a study of treatments performed at four general practitioners' offices and at a specialist clinic after 2 years. J Oral Rehabil 1995;22(8):543-8.

6.      Zoghbi SA, de Lima LA, Saraiva L, et al. Surgical experience influences 2-stage implant osseointegration. J Oral Maxillofac Surg 2011;69(11):2771- 6.

7.      Al-Sabbagh Mohanad, Bhavsar Ishita. Key Local and Surgical Factors Related to Implant Failure. Dent Clin N Am . 2015; (59)1-23.

8.      Lambert PM, Morris HF, Ochi S. Positive effect of surgical experience with implants on second-stage implant survival. J Oral Maxillofac Surg 1997;55(12 Suppl 5):12-8.

9.      Buser, D, Janne SFM, Wittneben JG, Bragger U, Ramseier CA, Salvi. GE. 10-Year Survival and Success Rates of 511 Titanium Implants with a Sandblasted and Acid-Etched Surface: A Retrospective Study in 303 Partially Edentulous Patients. Clinical Implant Dentistry and Related Research 2012. 14(6): 839-851.

10.     Noia CF, Ortega-Lopes R, Moraes M, Albergària-Barbosa JR, Moreira RWF, Mazzonetto R Rev Assoc Paul Cir Dent 2010;64(1):55-58.

11.     Silva AC, Campos AC, Moreira RWF. Analysis of intercurrences and complications in the installation of dental implants - a retrospective study. Rev. Cir. Traumatol. Camaragibe. 2010; 4 (10): 63-78.

12.     Bjarni P, Zwahlen AA, Irena MS Improvements in implant dentistry over the last decade: comparison of survival and complication rates in older and newer publications. International Journal of oral & Maxillofacial Implants. 2014; (29) 308-24.

13.     Ramalho-Ferreira G, Faverani LP, Gomes PCM, Assunçâo WG, Garcia Jùnior IR. Revista Odontológica de Araçatuba. 2010 31 (1): 51 -55.

14.     Pingarrón ML, Moràn MJ, Sànchez BR, Burgueno GM. Bronchial impaction of an implant screwdriver after accidental aspiration: report of a case and revision of the literature.

Oral Maxillofac Surg. 2010;14(1):43-7.

15.    Albuquerque, A. F. M., Cardoso, I. M. L., Silva, J. S. P. D., Germano, A. R., Dantas, W. R. M., & Gondim, A. L. M. F. Maxillary sinus lift using freeze-dried bone associated with immediate installation of a Morse cone implant: case report. *RFO UPF* .2014;19.(1): 129-134.

16.    Silva FC, Rebellatoll NLB, Fernandes A Implant planning in an atrophic maxilla: cone beam computed tomography case report. Rev. Cir. Traumatol. Buco-Maxilo-fac. 2013; 13(1):65-70.

17.    Misch CE, Resnik R. Mandibular nerve neurosensory impairment after dental implant surgery: management and protocol. Implant Dent. 2010;19(5):378-86.

18.    Santos PL, Germano EJ, Mattos JMB, Kuabara MR, Ferreira EJ, Gulinelli JL. Mandibular fracture after implant installation - case report. Full dent. Sci. 2015; 6(22):187-193.

19.    Dubois L, Lange J, Baas E, Van Ingen J. Excessive bleeding in the floor of the mouth after endosseous implant placement: a report of two cases. Int J Oral Maxillofac Surg. 2010;39(4):412-5.

20.    Dreiseidler T, Scherer P, Ketterle M, et al. Evaluation of maxillary sinus anatomy by conebeam CT prior to sinus floor elevation. Int J Oral Maxillofac Implants. 2010;25(2):258-65.

21.    Barros MCS, Cral WG, Rubira-Bullen ZRF, Capelozza ALA. Use and advantages of Cone-Beam Computed Tomography at a Public University. Rev Assoc Paul Cir Dent 2015; 69(4):336-9.

22.    Pinto, AVS. Risk factors in osseointegrated implant therapy [Master's dissertation]. Sao Paulo (Brazil): Department of Implant Dentistry, Castelo Branco University; 2000.

23.    Pelayo JL, Diago MP, Bowen EM, Diago MP. Intraoperative complications in oral implantology. Med Oral Pathol Oral Cir Bucal 2008;13(4):239-43.

24.    Christovam MC, Moscatiello RA, Moscatiello RM, Moscatiello VAM, Marques DE, Rocha DM, Schwed FNF.Infection control in implant dentistry. Innov Implant J, Biomater Esthet. 2011; 6,(1): 49-55.

25.    Fernàndez AA, Tejedor B, Palacios ERG, Zorzano LAA.Periodontics and Osteointegration. ^What influence does the administration of antibiotics have on the placement of dental implants? Literature review 2013; 23(3):159-164.

26. Eriksson RA, Albrektsson T, Magnusson B. Assessment of bone viability after heat trauma. A histological, histochemical and vital microscopic study in the rabbit. Scand J Plast Reconstr Surg 1984; 18(3):261-8.

27. NeroALD, Gehrke AS, Bortoli Jr. N, Zanatta LC. Temperature during bone milling. Comparative study of irrigation techniques. Rev. Assoc. Paul. Cir. Dent 2012; 66 (2): 147-50.

28. Nemcovsky CE, Artzi Z. Comparative study of buccal dehiscence defects in immediate, delayed, and late maxillary implant placement with collagen membrane: clinical healing between placement and second-stage surgery. J Periodontol. 2002; 73:754- 61.

29. Feller C, Gorab R. Updating the dental clinic. Sao Paulo: Artes Médicas, 2000. In: Neves JB. Oral implantology, optimizing aesthetics; a soft and hard tissue approach. Belo Horizonte: Traccio Arte e Desing; 2002.

30. Smeke L, Queiróz S, Kfouri FA. Subcutaneous emphysema associated with the use of a high-rotation pen during graft removal - case report. Full Dent. Sci. 2015; 6(23):275-278.

31. ZavanelliRA, GuilhermeAS, CastroAT, FernandesJMA, PereiraRE, Garcia RR. Local and systemic factors related to patients that can affect osseointegration. RGO - Rev Gaùcha Odontol. 2011; 59(0):133-146.

32. Alves-Rezende MCR, Bertoz APM, Grandini CR, Louzada MJQ, Santos APS, Capalbo BC, Alves-Claro APR. Osseointegration of Implants Installed without Primary Stability: The Role of Fibrin and Calcium Phosphate-Based Materials. Arch Health Invest.2012;1(1): 33-40.

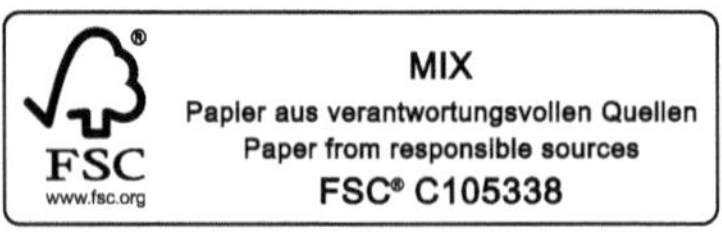


Printed by Books on Demand GmbH, Norderstedt / Germany